SMALLPOX

ADAM FURGANG

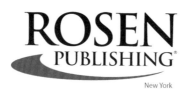

ROSEN
PUBLISHING®

New York

For all those throughout history taken by smallpox. And for Edward Jenner,
who saved countless generations

Published in 2011 by The Rosen Publishing Group, Inc.
29 East 21st Street, New York, NY 10010

Library of Congress Cataloging-in-Publication Data

Furgang, Adam.
Smallpox / Adam Furgang. — 1st ed.
     p. cm. — (Epidemics and society)
Includes bibliographical references and index.
ISBN 978-1-4358-9432-7 (library binding)
1. Smallpox—Popular works. I. Title.
RA644.S6F87 2011
614.5'21—dc22

                                                              2009046605

Manufactured in the United States of America

CPSIA Compliance Information: Batch #S10YA: For further information, contact Rosen Publishing, New York, New York, at
1-800-237-9932.

On the cover: the smallpox virus

CONTENTS

INTRODUCTION

O f all the diseases that humans have suffered throughout history, the biggest killer by far has been smallpox. It is believed that as many as half a billion people died from this disease in the twentieth century alone. Yet few people today even know what smallpox is and what its effects on the human body are. Now, the disease no longer exists as a threat to civilization. Modern medicine has helped wipe this disease off the face of the earth. Today, it only exists frozen in laboratories and does not affect humans anymore. It is no longer a threat to daily life and the way we live.

But smallpox was around for thousands of years before it was finally conquered. As it spread

4

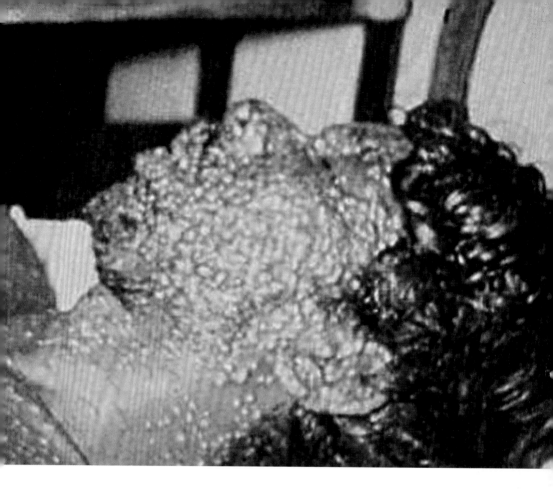

One of the symptoms of smallpox is the visually gruesome pox, or pustules, that cover a person's entire body, particularly the face.

throughout the world, it affected families, communities, and entire civilizations. It caused more deaths in the last hundred years than all the wars fought during that period combined. It influenced politics, affecting governments from one end of the earth to the other. The disease knew no economic, political, geographic, or social boundaries. It touched the lives of the rich and poor, kings and peasants, and chauffered presidents and ordinary pedestrians.

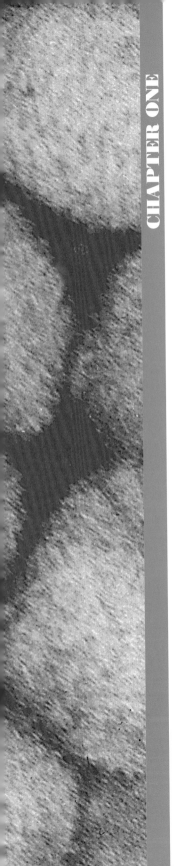

CHAPTER ONE

WHAT IS SMALLPOX?

One of the most devastating diseases to ever strike civilization is smallpox. It is an infection that is highly contagious, or easily spread from person to person. One of the most disturbing-looking and deadly symptoms of smallpox is the pustules, or pimplelike blisters, that cover the infected person's body.

Smallpox is caused by the variola virus. A virus is a microscopic agent that infects and replicates (makes copies of itself) in living cells. Many viruses can cause disease in the host. The severe blistering that smallpox causes is the reason the virus was named variola. The word comes from the Latin *varius,* meaning "spotted." The name "smallpox" was originally given to this disease so that people could tell it apart from another serious disease called syphilis. In its early stages, syphilis creates "large pox," or pustules, on a person's body. In England in the early 1500s, syphilis was often referred to as the "great pox."

The Spread of Smallpox

The exact origin of smallpox in humans is unclear. It is believed to have originated about

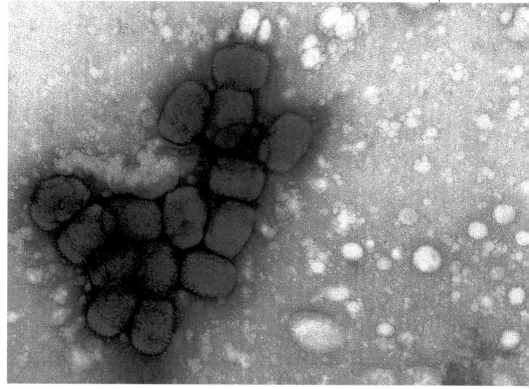

This is a transmission electron micrograph (TEM) of the smallpox virus cluster. Only with humanity's recent medical technology could the viruses be observed under microscopes. For much of history, humans did not even know viruses existed or what caused smallpox.

ten thousand years ago. This is when humans began farming in certain parts of the world and living in close quarters with animals, such as cows and camels.

The smallpox virus itself did not come directly from animals, but was passed in a similar form from animals to humans. Animals carry many viruses similar to the variola virus. Among them are the viruses commonly known as buffalo pox, camel pox, cowpox, crocodile pox, deer pox, monkey pox, rabbit pox, skunk pox, turkey pox, and vole pox. Once a form of pox virus was passed to humans, a genetic mutation, or change, likely occurred in the viral DNA that caused it to become deadly to humans. This deadly version, which is the variola virus that we know causes smallpox, only infects humans.

Smallpox spreads from human to human through the air via breathing, sneezing, or coughing. When a sick person

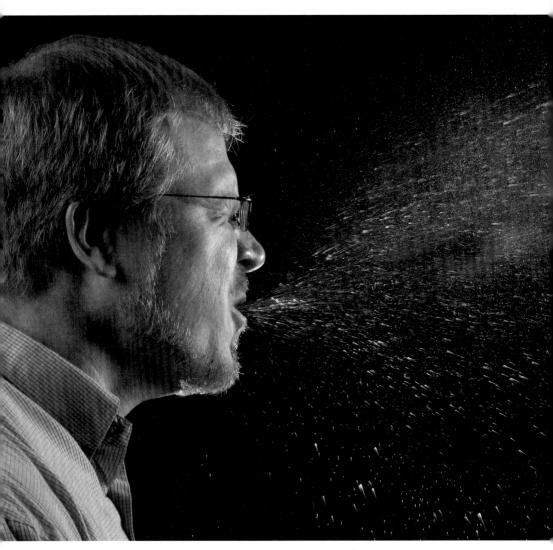

Smallpox and other diseases can spread easily from person to person through the air in salivary droplets when someone coughs or sneezes. This photo illustrates why it is important to cover one's mouth when coughing or sneezing.

infected with the disease coughs or sneezes, small droplets of fluid containing the variola virus are forced out into the air. These tiny droplets, too small to be seen, are then inhaled by a healthy person when he or she comes into contact with an

infected person. The virus can also be spread through contact with an infected person's bodily fluids or by touching items that person has contaminated.

The virus then begins to multiply and spread throughout the body, even before the newly infected person notices any symptoms. When variola is first contracted, it starts attacking the cells in the body. A single variola virus could use a single host human cell to produce as many as one hundred thousand copies of itself.

These copies of the original virus leave the infected cell by crossing the cell wall. Sometimes the release of these viral particles causes the infected cell to burst open, which kills the cell. After leaving the infected cell, these new viruses often infect other healthy cells that are nearby. This is how the virus spreads throughout the body. Eventually millions of previously healthy cells become infected. The spreading virus can then enter into the bloodstream and attack a person's organs, tissue, and skin. This puts a person's life at great risk.

The variola virus is rectangular in shape and measures roughly 0.000014 inches (350 nanometers) long. That may not sound big, but as viruses go, it is one of the biggest and hardiest. Its comparatively large size gives it the ability to protect itself better outside the human body when moving from host to host. It can also often survive outside a host over longer periods of time than smaller viruses.

Smallpox Symptoms

The variola virus spreads quietly throughout a person's body with no symptoms for the first ten to fourteen days. The

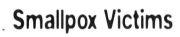

Smallpox Victims

Throughout history, billions of people suffered from smallpox. Some patients' faces became unrecognizable. Sometimes the skin would come off in sections. One of the more gruesome side effects of smallpox was the odor that could result from rotting flesh and cracking and oozing pustules. The smell could get so bad that patients died because people became afraid to tend to them or go near them.

Of those infected with smallpox, infants, pregnant women, the poor, the malnourished, and the elderly suffered the worst. Death rates for these groups tended to be high. Sometimes a malnourished person's eyes could be severely affected or even blinded. This was less common among victims who were healthy before becoming infected with the smallpox virus. Even the healthy that survived were still scarred. Telltale pockmark scars remained on people's faces and bodies for the rest of their lives.

disease spreads easiest once the infected person begins to show symptoms.

After about ten to twelve days, the infected person gets a high fever and body aches. This first sign of infection is often mistaken for the flu. However, the symptoms get worse. A rash begins to develop, accompanied by the first blisters or sores. Usually the back of a person's mouth and his or her nose and throat are affected early on. At this point, an infected person is extremely contagious because he or she begins coughing and sneezing. People who come in contact with an infected person are then at the greatest risk of catching the disease themselves. However, objects that the infected person has touched, such as clothing, sheets, and blankets, can also help spread the disease from person to person.

The sores then spread over a person's head, neck, and body. Meanwhile, the virus is busy attacking vital organs and inner tissue. Many of the body's inner membranes, which keep organs and tissues separate from one another, become affected. Internal bleeding may occur as the body is attacked from the inside. Some people's skin may turn dark red or black as a result. Bleeding can also occur from the eyes, mouth, and various other body openings. Death usually occurs far more quickly for patients who suffer from internal bleeding. And since a person with more densely clustered sores faces a 60 percent chance of death, it is usually a good sign when pustules occur less frequently on a person's body.

The pustules concentrate themselves in very sensitive areas of the body, causing extreme pain and discomfort for the infected. Most people suffer the largest concentration of sores on the hands, face, feet, neck, back, and arms. These sores can be very disfiguring.

After several weeks, those lucky enough to survive the horrible ordeal begin to get better. The high fever breaks and

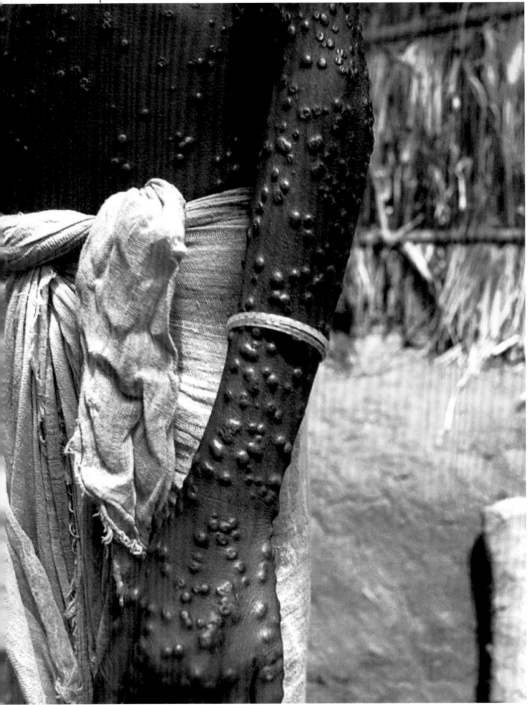

The unmistakable signs of smallpox are shown here on a boy from a Bangladesh village in 1974.

eventually the scabs that have formed over the sores begin to fall off. A person who survives smallpox is still contagious until the last scab has fallen off of his or her body (though the scabs themselves still contain viral particles that can infect healthy human cells). Most victims who survive the disease have permanent pockmarks, or scars, from the pustules that covered their skin.

If someone survives infection with the variola virus, the body's immune system can later recognize the virus and will not be infected or develop smallpox disease again.

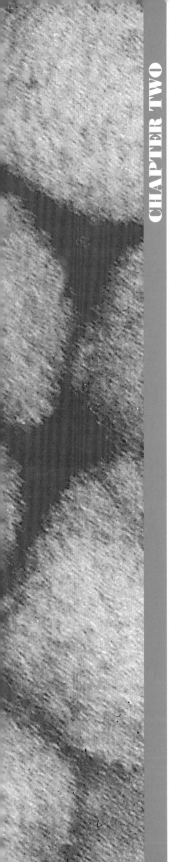

CHAPTER TWO

A BRIEF HISTORY OF SMALLPOX

Roughly ten thousand years ago, humans first developed simple agricultural and farming practices. Before that time, people hunted and gathered their food as they needed it. But humans eventually learned to use the land to plant or raise the food they needed in large quantities. Certain animals, such as cows, oxen, and horses, were used to move or carry heavy objects for humans. Cows, pigs, goats, and sheep were used for food, providing humans with milk and meat. All of these farm animals are called livestock.

Once humans began to produce food in this way, they began to live closer together and in larger, permanent communities. Communities massed around the agricultural centers, and people lived close by to help work on the farms. People also began to live and work closer to the animals that helped them farm or were raised for food. Domesticated animals were very important to these first farmers. They would work all day in close contact with their livestock in their constant effort to put food on the table and avoid poverty and starvation.

Animals, just like humans, have their own unique diseases and viruses that have evolved

14

over millions of years. It is very likely that living in close proximity to cows, horses, pigs, and sheep was the way smallpox moved from farm animals to humans. Although no one knows for sure, scientists think that some form of cowpox or a similar virus was passed to humans from the animals they lived and worked with. Some form of animal virus probably infected a person or group of people, and it was then passed on to other humans. Eventually, the virus mutated, or changed, into the variola virus. Today, we know this virus causes the disease smallpox, which is deadly only to humans.

Earliest Cases of Smallpox

How do scientists know how long smallpox has been around? Written or visual records of smallpox have been produced around the world for thousands of years. Written texts from Egypt dating to around 3000 BCE describe an illness that resembles smallpox. Records from the Indian subcontinent dating to 1500 BCE tell of smallpox arriving there, most likely from Egyptian traders. Some of these ancient documents include pictures that describe the visual symptoms of smallpox, while others reveal elaborate treatments to aid people with the disease.

The greatest evidence for smallpox's long history are the mummified remains of Pharaoh Ramses V of Egypt. His preserved head and upper body show scars that were likely caused by smallpox. He died around 1157 BCE, possibly from the disease.

The Romans were also likely victims of smallpox. Between 165 and 180 CE, Rome was hit with a mysterious epidemic, or widespread outbreak of disease. Historians call this epidemic the Plague of Antoninus. It likely killed 3.5

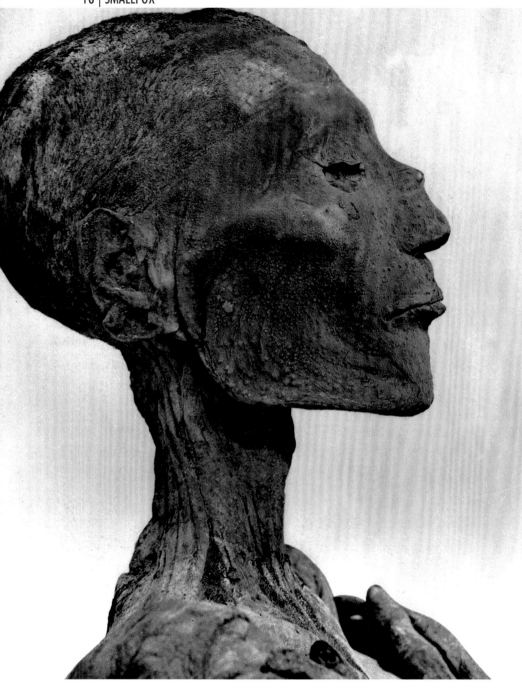

By examining the mummy of Pharaoh Ramses V of Egypt, it has been speculated that he probably died from smallpox. Scars can be seen on his neck and face, likely caused by smallpox. This is the earliest evidence of smallpox in history.

million to seven million people during this time. The epidemic was once widely believed to be smallpox, although some historians today feel that it may have been measles. Even so, all historians agree that smallpox was a deadly killer for thousands of years.

The Virus Arrives in the New World

It is likely that smallpox first passed from animals to humans in the Middle East, Africa, or Asia. From there, it spread to Europe. Eventually, smallpox became endemic to Europe. That means that it could be regularly and commonly found there.

In 1520, Spanish explorer Hernán Cortés arrived in Mexico. Traveling with Cortés and his crew was a slave who was infected with smallpox. This single infected person was enough to cause a massive smallpox epidemic among the native Aztec people. They had no immunity to the disease because they had never encountered it before. Their immune systems were wholly unprepared and unable to effectively fight the newly arrived virus. Mexico's original native population was around twenty million at the time the Spanish explorers arrived. By 1618, there were only around 1.6 million native peoples left.

Similar to this outbreak in Mexico, smallpox was spread among the Incas in South America by the Spanish in 1526. This epidemic ultimately killed a large portion of the Incan population. Even the Inca's emperor, Huayna Capac, was killed by this devastating disease.

When the first settlers came to the New World, they not only brought new technologies, such as guns, but also their deadly diseases. It was the diseases from Europe, especially smallpox, that had the most devastating effect on the native peoples of the New World. Far more of North and South

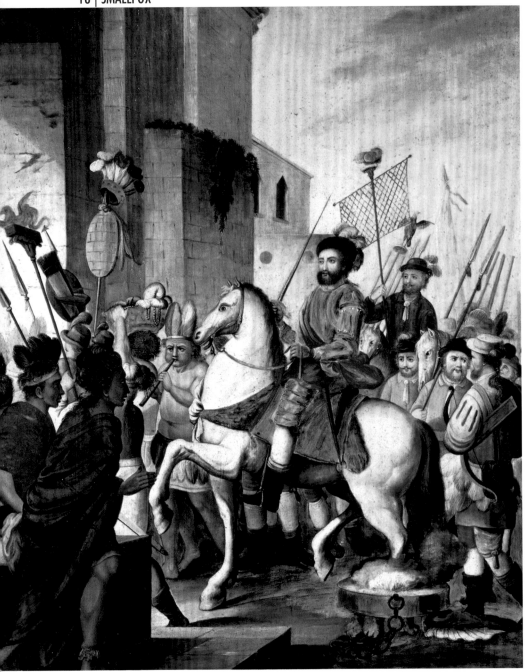

The Spanish conquistador Hernán Cortés invades Mexico in 1519. The diseases his forces brought with them did more to harm the native populations than the violent warfare they waged.

America's native population were killed by disease than by the colonial wars of conquest that eventually took place.

Native American Vulnerability to Smallpox

At the time settlers came to the New World, the virus that causes smallpox was not yet endemic to North America and South America. That means that the native people there had little immunity to the virus. Immunity is the ability of an organism to fight or resist an infection. Smallpox had already been with the Europeans for centuries, so many of the settlers in the New World had already been exposed to the variola virus in their original countries. This meant that the European survivors of smallpox were protected from future infection. When the variola virus began to spread in the Americas, it was the native populations that suffered far more from smallpox than did the Europeans. Every Native American was able to be infected with the virus and develop the disease, whereas a much smaller percentage of the Europeans were able to be infected.

Not all Europeans had become immune to the smallpox virus, however. More than forty thousand people a year were killed by the disease in eighteenth-century Europe alone. In the early American settlements and the later colonies, smallpox was still a grave threat to these growing populations.

Smallpox at Plymouth Plantation

Smallpox came to the New World with the earliest explorers and European settlers. In 1617, a few years before the Pilgrims landed in what would become Plymouth, Massachusetts, a smallpox epidemic swept through the Massachusetts coastal areas. Within two years, 90 percent of the Native Americans who became infected with the virus died from smallpox. Tribes such as the Massachuset, the Wampanoag, and the Pawtucket were virtually wiped out by the epidemic.

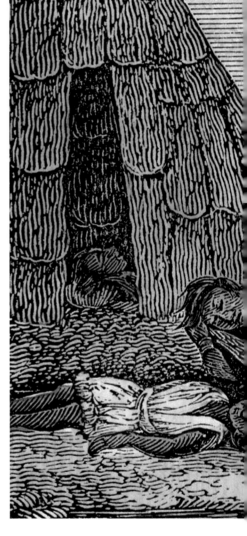

In 1620, Pilgrims landed in Plymouth. In succeeding years, large numbers of English settlers continued to arrive in Massachusetts. These settlers, known as the Puritans, came to the New World searching for religious freedom. In 1633, another smallpox epidemic hit Massachusetts, wiping out large numbers of Native Americans. During this epidemic, only twenty Plymouth colonists contracted smallpox.

Some Puritans saw this epidemic as a gift from their God, showing his favor toward them and his displeasure with the Native Americans. One of the first presidents of Harvard College, a clergyman named Increase Mather, had this to say about the epidemic: "The Indians began to be quarrelsome concerning the bounds of the land they had sold to the English; but God ended the controversy by sending the smallpox amongst the

Indians at Saugust, who were before that time exceeding numerous. Whole towns of them were swept away, in some of them not so much as one soul escaping the destruction" (as quoted by Ian and Jenifer Glynn in *The Life and Death of Smallpox*).

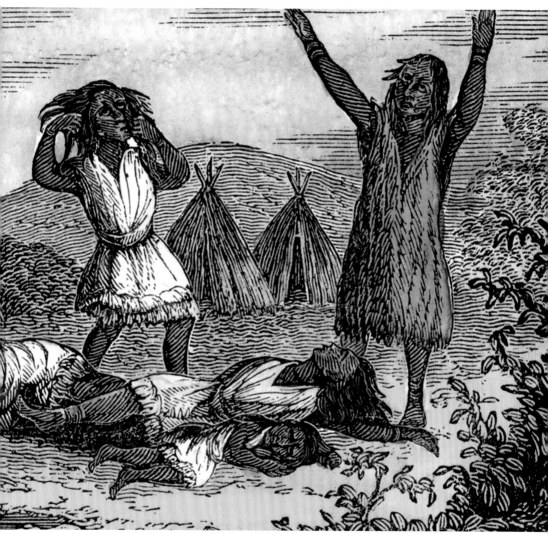

When European settlers came to the New World, they brought smallpox with them. Native Americans had not been exposed to this disease, so they had no immunity to it and were devastated by its effects.

Smallpox and the American Revolution

Before and during the time of the American Revolution, smallpox was used as a weapon of war. In 1763, Native Americans threatened Fort Pitt in Pennsylvania. In response, the British gave two blankets and one handkerchief to Native Americans and an Ottawa leader named Chief Pontiac as "gifts." These items had been deliberately taken from a smallpox hospital with the purpose of infecting and killing the Native Americans.

During the American Revolution, a huge epidemic of smallpox killed more Americans than did the war itself. Rumors of the British using smallpox as an early form of germ warfare had the American soldiers and colonists living in fear.

Smallpox and the Slave Trade

The slave trade was another way that diseases spread from one country to another and from one continent to another. Smallpox had arrived in Mexico and killed millions. The epidemic was traced back to a single infected slave who had come from Spanish Cuba.

During the time of the American slave trade, smallpox was a serious problem in the Americas. Slave owners needed to be assured that their new slaves were disease-free. News advertisements and printed flyers of the time boasted that slaves from specific ships had already survived smallpox in their native lands and were now immune to infection. Claims were also made that slaves for sale had been kept free from infected areas and were therefore "clean." This made buying from certain slave traders more attractive. Still, slaves were often transported in unsanitary conditions on densely crowded ships, and some died of smallpox and other diseases before ever reaching the Americas.

These rumors were so serious that people such as General George Washington and president of the Continental Congress John Hancock discussed the problem in the Massachusetts House of Representatives. They feared that if the epidemic hit the American troops, their chances of winning the war would be ruined.

It is hard to know whether a naturally occurring epidemic or human-engineered germ warfare was responsible for the death of so many Americans during the Revolution. But the constant threat of smallpox epidemics kept civilizations all around the world in a state of fear and great danger well into the twentieth century.

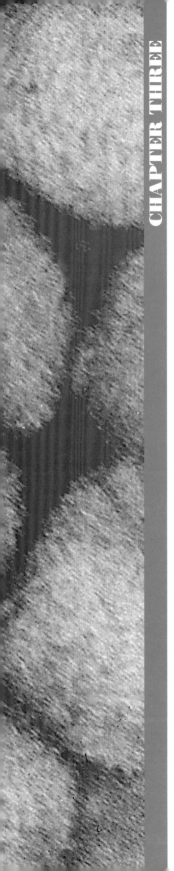

CHAPTER THREE

EARLY TREATMENTS

Smallpox existed long before people had accurate and reliable knowledge of medicine and how diseases spread. It was thousands of years before people could understand smallpox and explain what caused it. One early theory was that smallpox was due to an imbalance within the victims' bodies. Other theories blamed toxic gases seeping from the ground. Still others believed the disease was a result of God's anger. For example, in China, Africa, India, and, later, South America, people worshiped gods or goddesses associated with smallpox. Sometimes sacrifices were made to these gods to keep them from striking down more victims of the disease.

It was perhaps even more difficult for people to treat smallpox than it was for them to understand it. Throughout history, people have made many attempts to cure this deadly disease. Many of the therapies and "remedies" seem gruesome by the standards of modern medical treatments.

Early Therapies

One arcane method of treating smallpox victims was the bleeding of the patient. People's bodies

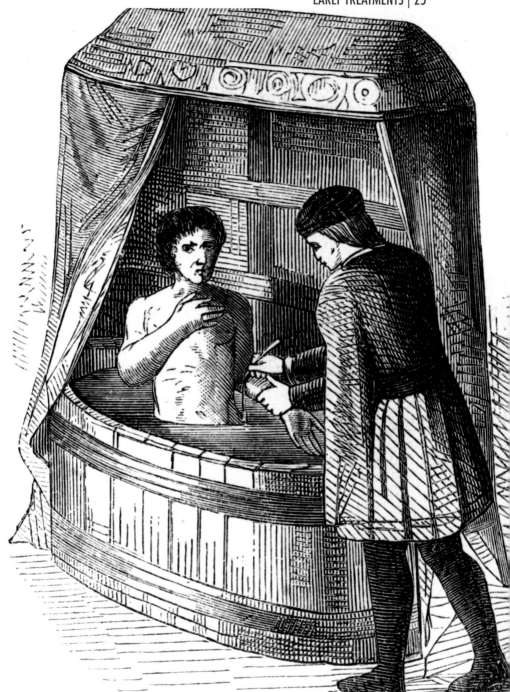

Ignorant to the real causes of the disease, some early treatments did more harm than good. In the treatment shown here, blood is being drained from the patient's body to get rid of the disease.

would be "bled," or drained of their blood, often to the point where the patient would faint. It was believed that this would help remove the disease from the patient.

Horrible combinations of substances, or tonics, were also given to people with smallpox to help rid them of the disease. Mixtures of powdered horse dung, lye, mouse whiskers, and crumbled sponges were among the ingredients in some smallpox tonics. Putting a cloth drenched in vinegar under the patient's nose or placing a bag of camphor around the patient's neck was also an early attempt to cure the disease.

Heat therapy and red therapy were also quite common. Because smallpox caused high fevers in patients, it was thought that exposing the patients to heat might draw the fever out and rid them of the disease. This practice was not just a home remedy of the times. It was also used by doctors. They would cover patients in heavy wool blankets and then put them near a huge fire, even in the heat of summer.

The color red is associated with heat as well as with the physical effects of smallpox, especially the tell-tale blisters. These color associations are what inspired red therapy. Patients were dressed in red, surrounded by red cloths, placed in red rooms, and even fed red liquids or juices made from red berries.

Many people died, not from smallpox, but rather from the extreme and ineffective treatments of the times. These treatments did not help the patients and only added to their suffering, further draining their bodies' strength just when it was needed most.

Small Steps Forward

Around the year 950 CE, a very important observation was made about smallpox that helped people understand it a little

Smallpox Vaccines

Smallpox vaccines are 95 percent effective in preventing the disease. The vaccine lasts for three to five years, and then a person's immunity to the disease begins to lessen. After that time, a person must be vaccinated again to continue immunity. Once a person gets infected with the smallpox virus, it is still not too late to be vaccinated. He or she can receive a vaccine within a few days of exposure. This late vaccination can still prevent the disease or lessen its effects.

The vaccine is usually given in the upper arm in the form of several small pricks with a two-pronged needle that has droplets of the vaccine on it. Within a few days, itchy red bumps form at the site of the vaccination. Within several weeks, the bumps become blisters that fill with pus and drain. Finally, scabs form and then fall off. When a person is revaccinated, the side effects are not as severe as they were the first time.

better. People began to realize that when someone had small-pox and survived, they did not develop the disease again. Something changed in the body of a smallpox survivor. It was not yet clear to people what exactly had changed, but it was under-stood that a person could not catch the disease twice. Doctors of that time did not know what we know now about the body's immune system. Once the body survives the variola virus, even a mild case, the immune system knows how to defeat that particular virus and will not be infected again.

In China, a technique was developed that used this knowledge to prevent people from getting the disease in the first place. The smallpox scabs from a survivor were ground up into a powder or dust. Healthy people who had never had smallpox inhaled this powder through their noses. People who underwent this new technique, called variolation, would get a mild form of smallpox. They would experience fever, rash, and pustules, but then become better. Similar forms of the technique appeared in India and Africa.

As this method of disease prevention spread, the technique became more refined. By the end of the 1600s, the knowledge had spread across Asia and into the Turkish Empire. By then, powder from dried scabs was no longer being inhaled. Instead, tiny drops of pus were taken from the pustules of people who had mild cases of smallpox. The pus was inserted under the skin of healthy people, which caused a mild case of the disease. This idea of introducing a small amount of a virus into a person's body to create immunity against a full-blown case of the disease eventually became known as inoculation.

Inoculation had some positive and negative effects. While it kept people from getting a full-blown case of smallpox during an epidemic, it still gave them a mild case of the disease. About 1 or 2 percent of people inoculated died from the inoculation. The biggest drawback, however, was that coming into contact with a person who was mildly sick from inoculation could spread the full-blown form of the disease. This meant that healthy people were giving themselves a mild form of the disease while perhaps spreading more severe and life-threatening cases of it.

A Clue Found Among Milkmaids

The eventual cure for smallpox can be credited to a small-town doctor from England. In the late 1700s, a man named Edward Jenner found a way to prevent smallpox without the side effects of inoculation. Jenner trained as a surgeon and spent time as

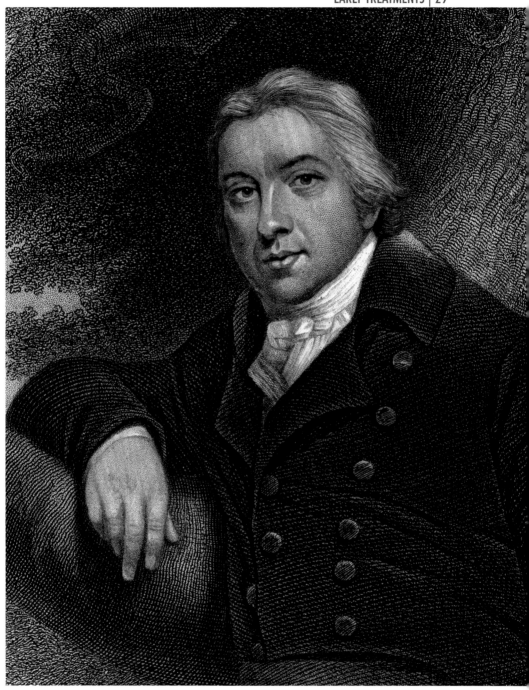

Edward Jenner's discovery and development of the smallpox vaccine
ended up saving the lives of millions of people around the world.

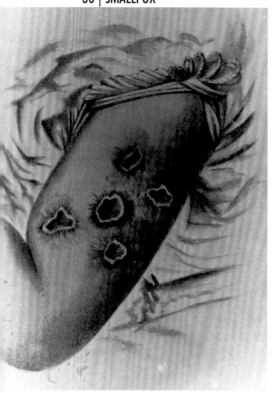

This illustration shows the arm of a young girl eight days after being vaccinated by Edward Jenner's cowpox vaccine.

a doctor in the town in which he had grown up. Over time, he noticed that milkmaids who had been exposed to cows and a disease called cowpox did not come down with smallpox. His observation was dismissed by his peers, and he did not try to prove his theory until years later.

During the next smallpox outbreak that hit his town, Jenner again observed that milkmaids who had gotten cowpox remained unaffected by smallpox. The milkmaids were contracting cowpox from pustules on the cows' udders, perhaps through small scrapes on their hands or by touching or rubbing their own eyes after milking the cows. The milkmaids came down with a disease similar to that of people inoculated against smallpox. The only difference was that their cases were far less severe. Cowpox symptoms were akin to a severe cold, nothing more. Most important, cowpox did not kill the animals or the people who were infected with it. The milkmaids were never covered in pustules or scarred by the pox sores. As a result of not getting pox or scarring, milkmaids were long celebrated for the beauty of their clear, smooth skin.

In 1796, Jenner conducted the first of his famous experiments in which he inserted the pus from a cowpox pustule into a healthy person. His first experiment was on an eight-year-old boy. He inserted the pus into an incision in the boy's arm. This gave the boy an immunity to smallpox, and it proved Jenner's theory. Being able to eliminate the dangerous practice of smallpox inoculation and replace it with the far less dangerous cowpox inoculation was a huge step in medicine. It was also a giant leap forward for the health and well-being of the entire world.

However, Jenner's ideas and experiments were met with criticism. Some believed he needed to present further proof of the cowpox inoculation's effectiveness against smallpox

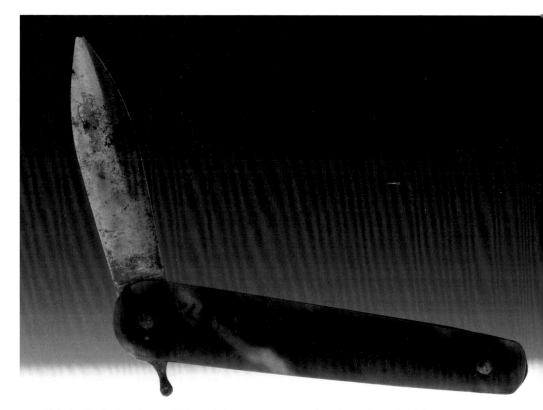

This knife, belonging to Edward Jenner, was used to introduce fluid from a cowpox sore into the body of a healthy person. This was one of the earliest forms of vaccination.

infection. So Jenner conducted the experiments on even more people. Eventually, the medical and scientific community accepted Jenner's theory, and his technique spread and was further perfected.

Vaccination

Jenner called the cowpox inoculation a vaccination, after the Latin word *vacca*, meaning "cow." That term is still used today when a weakened form of a virus is given to someone to provide immunity against that virus. Jenner ultimately became one of the most well-respected doctors in the world. He is known today as the Father of Immunology.

Jenner's revolutionary ideas led the fight to produce vaccines against many other illnesses that have plagued civilization. Measles, chicken pox, mumps, typhoid, bubonic plague, influenza, typhoid, and hepatitis B are some of the infectious diseases that are prevented by vaccines. There is no question of the positive and lifesaving effects vaccines have had on humanity as a whole. Millions of people who are alive today would surely have died from various diseases and illnesses were it not for Jenner's important discovery. In fact, there are no remaining cases of smallpox in the world. Thanks to vaccination, the disease has been completely eradicated, or wiped out, and is no longer a threat to humanity.

CHAPTER FOUR

FAMILIES IN ISOLATION

"No man dares count his children as his own until after they have had smallpox." This proverb shows just how common and deadly smallpox was in the past. Today, it is hard to understand how something so horrible and devastating could also be so common.

Isolation

For thousands of years, smallpox had a profound effect on the family. A deadly scourge that was not contained until the beginning of the twentieth century, the disease affected families from all countries, whether they were rich or poor. However, smallpox hit poor families most severely because they tended to be malnourished. People who are malnourished have a weaker immune system, which makes it harder for them to cope with the harsh effects of disease.

Once smallpox struck within a house, an enormous and often deadly strain was placed upon the family. Many families were forced to live in close quarters with ill and contagious brothers, sisters, mothers, or fathers. Once people learned that smallpox spread from person to person through physical contact, isolation

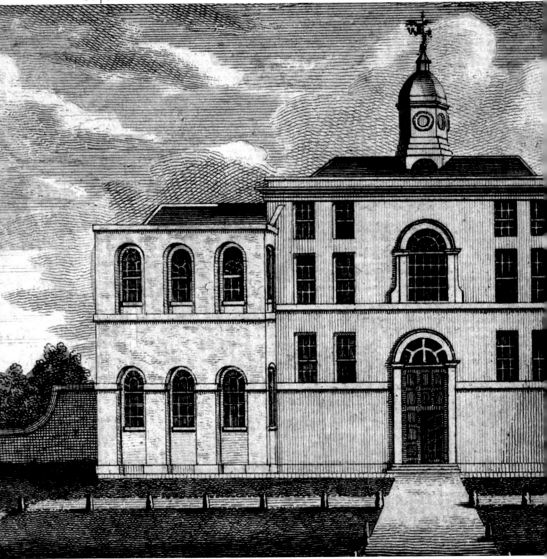

The St. Pancras Smallpox Inoculation Hospital in London, England, appears above in a c. 1800 print. This institution was devoted to the inoculation of the poor against smallpox.

became an important way to treat family members without spreading the disease. The period of time a contagious person is placed in isolation during a disease outbreak is called quarantine.

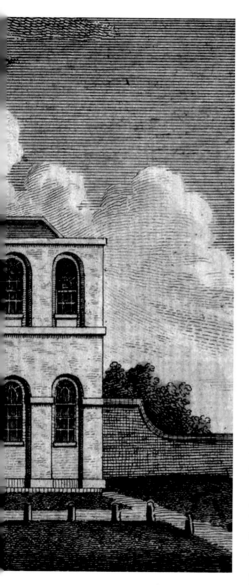

To many families, putting their loved ones in quarantine was the only way to keep other family members from catching the disease. However, some isolated their loved ones in a very harsh way. Sometimes people simply abandoned ill family members in the woods and left them to die. Some people, terrified by the prospect of deadly illness raging through an entire family, felt forced to abandon children, spouses, or parents.

Rich Family, Poor Family: Inoculation and Class

Before Edward Jenner discovered the process of smallpox vaccination using the mild cowpox virus, the only protection people had against smallpox was variolation. This was inoculation with the smallpox virus itself. This process was very dangerous and controversial. It could also spread smallpox at its fullest strength. Still, many families feared smallpox so much that they took the risk and had their entire families inoculated. They felt that full-blown smallpox infection posed a greater risk than variolation.

Smallpox Island

In 1647, a smallpox outbreak in the Massachusetts colony caused leaders to start a quarantine in order to separate the sick from the healthy. An act was also passed requiring that a red flag be flown outside any household infected with smallpox. Other areas of colonial America required households to post notices warning would-be visitors that a person in the home suffered from smallpox. Guards were even used to turn people away from some homes where family members had smallpox. In the colony of Rhode Island, an island called Coasters Harbor Island was used to quarantine people. The island soon was referred to as Smallpox Island.

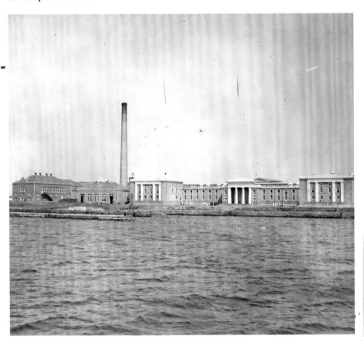

Coasters Harbor Island, off the coast of Rhode Island, was the site of a smallpox quarantine hospital in the eighteenth century. The site was later used as the Newport Asylum for the Poor and, starting in 1882, by the Navy for its Naval War College, which still operates there today.

However, the process of variation angered many poor families because they could not afford it. They felt this put them at greater risk of getting smallpox than members of wealthier families. Even families that could afford to pay for the procedure often could not afford to miss the pay they would lose from being out of work while ill after the procedure. People would be sick for up to four weeks while they suffered from the weakened form of the smallpox virus received during variolation.

Smallpox and its treatment and prevention soon exposed class strains in colonial America. In 1774, two inoculation hospitals opened in Salem and Marblehead, Massachusetts. Angry citizens, unable to afford variolation, destroyed one of the hospitals, and both were eventually closed. That same year, a smallpox epidemic hit Philadelphia, Pennsylvania, killing more than three hundred people, mostly children from poor families. Because wealthy families often employed workers in their homes, the virus spread to the poorer workers from their employers who had undergone and were protected by variolation.

Outbreaks and the Strain Placed on Families

Smallpox outbreaks struck crowded European cities differently than they did the newly settled and sparsely populated American colonies. European cities barely saw a pause between outbreaks of the disease. It passed more or less continuously through families and communities without stopping.

In North America, however, because it was easier to keep people isolated and thus stop the disease, the outbreaks seemed to come roughly every five years. But each time a new outbreak occurred, the virus caused disease and death among a new set of people, both children and adults alike. By the time the next round of disease arrived, there was a new group of people who had already survived smallpox and were now immune to it. Yet there would also be a new group of children under the age of five who had not yet been born when the last outbreak occurred. They were much more susceptible to infection than their other family members. That is why the disease affected so many more young people than it did adults.

Although families may have had members who gained immunity to smallpox because they had it when they were younger, the effects on the family were still great. The healthy were left to care for the sick, often missing work and losing income as a result. They also had to bear the emotional burden of isolating their sick family members from others.

Many families in Europe, as well as the Americas, relied on the labor of every family member to help make ends meet. For example, children worked in fields, tending to crops and feeding animals. When infection struck down family members, it was hard to do the work the sick person once did, whether it was farming, running a store, or manufacturing or trading goods. It could quickly become difficult for these families to put food on the table. Healthy family members could easily become worn down and overworked while

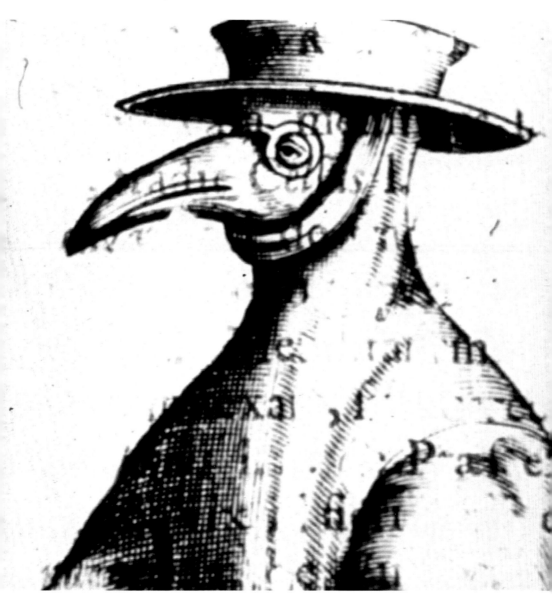

During the seventeenth century, doctors wore protective masks and costumes like this to avoid infection while seeing patients.

trying to make up the extra workload. These people could become weakened and sick as well, even if they did not contract smallpox. They could become vulnerable to other illnesses and diseases.

Communities often viewed infected families as people to stay away from—to "avoid like the plague"—rather than as a group of individuals who required lifesaving help and compassion. When a colonial family placed a red flag in front of their home, it did more than just inform their neighbors of smallpox infection on the premises. It isolated the family from the community. People did not offer help, but left families to their own devices to suffer or die from the deadly disease.

COMMUNITIES BESIEGED

Smallpox has been affecting communities large and small for thousands of years. When the disease first began to affect small communities of farmers thousands of years ago, people did not know what was happening. They did not realize what caused the disease and how and where they may have been exposed to it.

For the smallpox virus to continue to exist, it needs a large enough population to keep it going. In ancient communities that were too small or too far apart from each other, smallpox would have killed its victims and simply died out before the virus reached another small and distant community. But larger and closer communities allowed the variola virus to spread. The more people in a community, the more hosts the virus could find to live in and infect.

When communities became more interconnected through trade and travel, the smallpox virus could travel via hosts to new places and infect whole new groups of people. As farmers and tradespeople moved from place to place to trade goods, the disease was passed to new communities. As greater trading between Asia, North Africa, and Europe

41

developed, smallpox was beginning to spread throughout the known world.

From 165 to 180 CE, smallpox hit Rome and started what is now called the Plague of Antoninus. This was one of

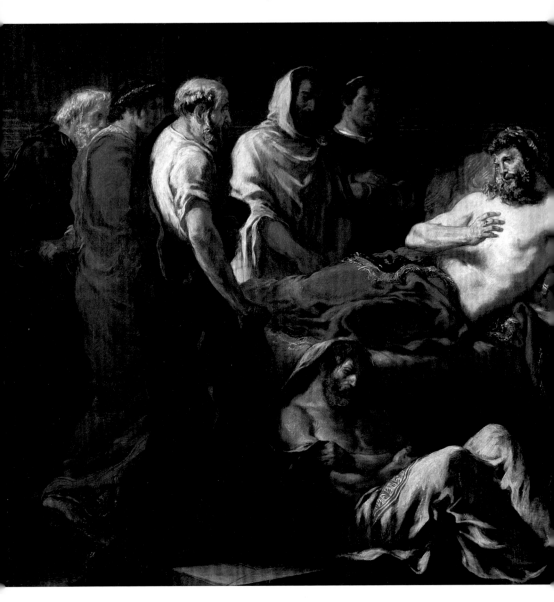

This study for the painting *The Death of Marcus Aurelius* was painted by Eugene Delacroix. It depicts the plague that hit Rome from 165 to 180 CE.

the world's largest population centers at the time. Millions of citizens in Rome were killed by this plague. Some estimates place those killed by the epidemic at between 3.5 to 7 million people. Even the Roman emperor Marcus Aurelius was killed.

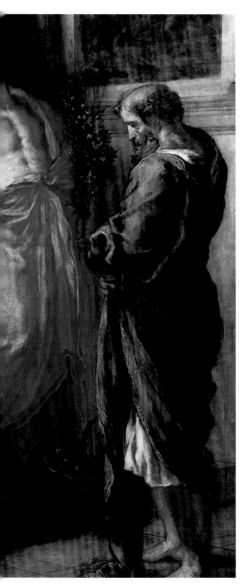

Panic in the Streets

When epidemics hit communities today, people usually act quickly in order to protect themselves, help each other, and stop the spread of the disease. Today, health emergencies in a community can bring people together. This was not the case hundreds of years ago. Once people knew that smallpox was passed by person-to-person contact, the first appearance of an outbreak terrified community members. In effect, smallpox victims were disowned by their communities, and sometimes even by their own families. People feared getting the disease themselves and dying from it. Community members did not rush to help each other because they knew the disease might kill the victims, whether they were given help or not. And in giving help, they might expose themselves to infection, illness, and death.

The fear of spreading the disease was a real one. But the fear was so great that, in 1803, a special law was passed by the governor of Bohemia (the modern-day Czech Republic). This law prevented people from attending the funerals of smallpox victims. Even family members and clergy were forbidden to go to the burials for fear that the disease could be passed from the dead victim to the funeral goers. We now know that this isn't possible, but people lived in great fear of this seemingly uncontrollable and invincible killer.

Closed for Business

Communities could be torn apart by smallpox outbreaks. In the nineteenth and early twentieth centuries, communities were heavily dependent upon the laborers, factory workers, craftsmen, freight haulers, shop employees, and merchants who kept the wheels of commerce oiled and spinning. During smallpox outbreaks, many businesses could not continue as usual. Storeowners and tradespeople may have become ill themselves or had to close their businesses to care for loved ones. A person might find that the only store where they could buy cloth, food, or other goods was suddenly closed. The only blacksmith, post office, or bank in town might suddenly be shuttered. There could be no telling when the business might open again, if at all.

During smallpox outbreaks, many people feared going out in public at all. Businesses that remained open suffered because there were fewer customers willing to go out into the streets and mingle with crowds. Public gatherings were often discouraged or outlawed, and theater and concert performances were cancelled. Friends stopped visiting each other or meeting for dinner in restaurants. The social, civic, and cultural life of communities withered during smallpox epidemics. Life during

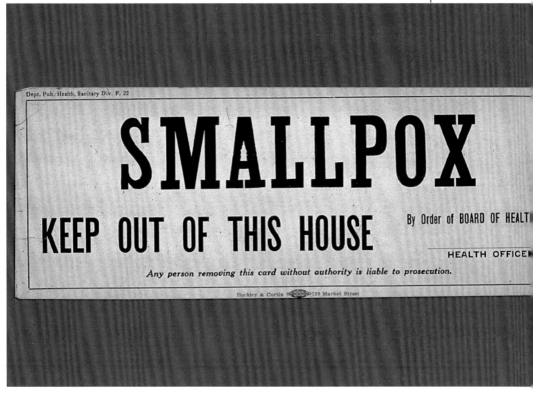

Dept. Pub./Health, Sanitary Div. F. 22

SMALLPOX

KEEP OUT OF THIS HOUSE

By Order of BOARD OF HEALTH

HEALTH OFFICE

Any person removing this card without authority is liable to prosecution.

Buckley & Curtin 739 Market Street

When a family member suffered from smallpox, the family was given a sign to place outside their home so that others would stay away.

an epidemic was definitely not the same as during times when smallpox was not a threat. People lived in constant fear.

Smallpox Hospitals

Some of the bravest people in the fight against smallpox were those who worked in smallpox hospitals. These were people who had survived the disease themselves or had been inoculated through variolation. They cared for the sick and either nursed them back to health or compassionately tended to those who were dying. Most communities were not lucky enough to have a smallpox hospital. Bringing a sick patient a far distance to a smallpox hospital was often too great a strain on the patient. Instead, some families living far from help were forced to quarantine or isolate their family members on their own.

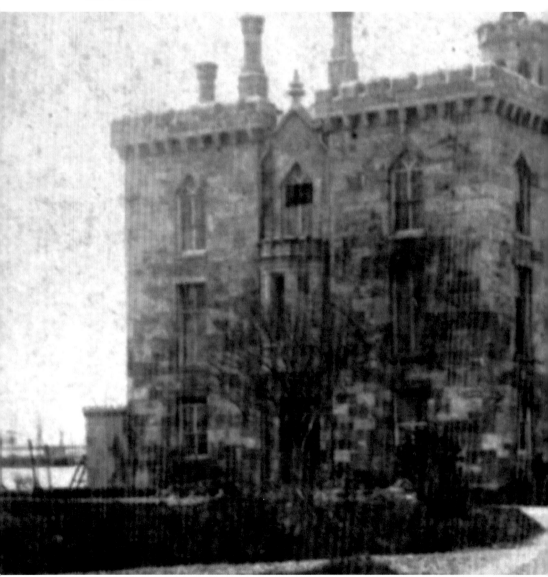

This smallpox hospital on Roosevelt Island in New York City opened in 1856. It had rooms for one hundred patients.

In large, densely populated communities like New York City, it was difficult to control and contain smallpox. For many years, the city kept sufferers separated from the rest of the community by putting them in wooden shacks along the East

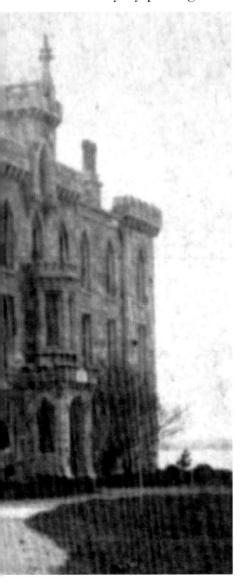

River. In 1856, the Smallpox Hospital was opened on Roosevelt Island (then known as Blackwell's Island and later as Welfare Island). Roosevelt Island is a small island in the middle of the East River, between Manhattan Island and Queens. The hospital was the first one in the country that was devoted exclusively to the care of people with infectious diseases. It was also the only hospital in New York City where a person with smallpox could go for treatment.

The hospital had room for one hundred patients, and it was the city's way of treating smallpox victims with care and compassion. The building was designed by the same architect who built New York City's famed Saint Patrick's Cathedral. After smallpox was eradicated in the United States, the Roosevelt Island hospital became a nurses' hospital. It was abandoned in the 1950s and lies in ruins today.

Myths and Facts

MYTH Smallpox symptoms show up soon after infection.

FACT There is an incubation period lasting from seven to seventeen days during which an infected person may show no symptoms and feel fine.

MYTH Smallpox is highly infectious, and one person can infect dozens of people through casual contact.

FACT Smallpox is contagious, but not highly contagious. It is not spread by casual or brief contact, but by close, intimate, or household contact. Generally, at least three hours of face-to-face contact is necessary to spread the virus. Ordinarily, one infected person who is not quarantined spreads the virus to no more than five or six other people. Measles and the flu are more contagious than smallpox.

MYTH The smallpox vaccine will not protect the patient who is already exposed to the variola virus.

FACT If a person is vaccinated within three days of exposure, smallpox will be completely prevented or its severity will be greatly reduced. Vaccination within four to seven days of exposure to the variola virus still offers some protection from the disease or may lessen the severity of it.

GOVERNMENTS UNDER ATTACK

When we consider the profound effect small-pox had on civilization, we realize just how much the disease has changed the world. It affected more than just families and communities. Smallpox epidemics even "infected" world politics and governments.

In Europe, before the New World had even been explored, smallpox was already changing the course of history. The disease was passed from the Eastern world to the Western world as the two sides warred during the Crusades. During the eleventh and fourteenth centuries, Christians tried to win the biblical Holy Land, including Jerusalem, back from the Muslims. Smallpox outbreaks occurred during this time. As a result, the disease spread from the Middle East into Europe and, from there, throughout the world during the Age of Exploration. The disease did not even spare royalty. In 1368, Prince John, son of King Edward the II of England, came down with smallpox.

An Empire Slayer

Smallpox destroyed entire civilizations. The Aztec and the Incan empires were wiped out

49

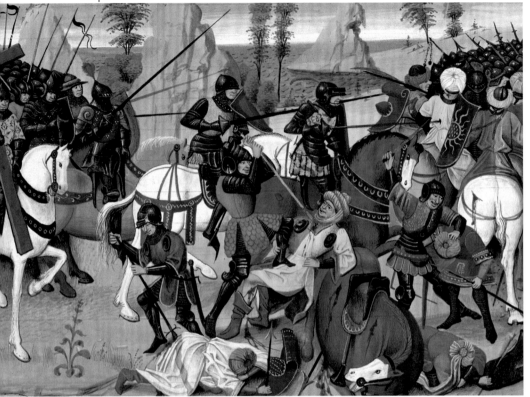

This illuminated image from 1462 shows a twelfth-century battle between the French forces of King Baldwin I and Turks during the long series of wars known as the Crusades.

within only a few generations of the arrival of the Europeans. It wasn't only weapons and bloodshed that destroyed these advanced civilizations. Smallpox killed far more people in both of those empires than did war. As a result, Europeans had far less trouble settling the area than they would have if the disease had not been present among the native peoples.

To give an idea of how deadly smallpox was, some historians estimate that when European explorers first came to the New World, there were more people living in the Americas than in Europe. That quickly changed as the Europeans introduced smallpox to this part of the world and the Native American population dwindled dramatically.

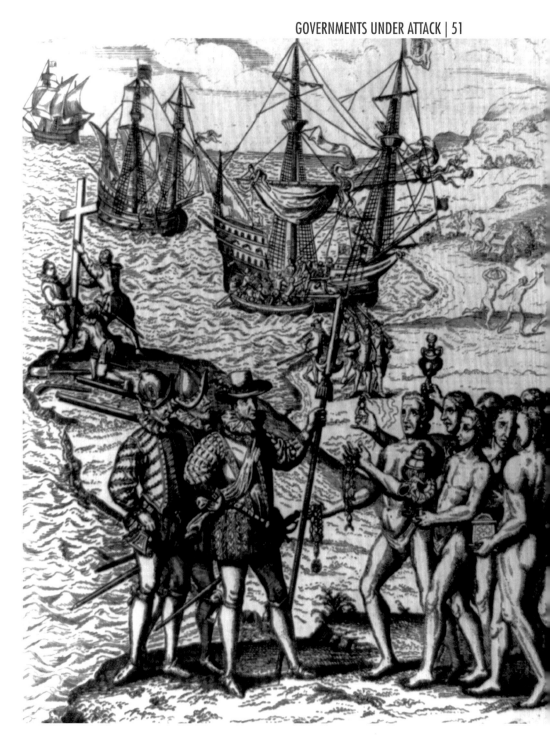

This print shows the moment Christopher Columbus first made contact with native inhabitants of the New World on the island of Hispaniola (which contains both Haiti and the Dominican Republic).

In 1492, when Christopher Columbus first reached what is now called the Dominican Republic, there were around a million native peoples living there. By 1620, none were left alive. Smallpox was the biggest reason for this tremendously fast decline. Just imagine how different the historical outcome might have been if smallpox had not been introduced to a population with no immunity to the disease. The Spanish would have had much more difficulty colonizing Mexico by waging war against the millions of native inhabitants who did not want them there. Smallpox changed history by making it much easier for settlers from the Old World to colonize the New World and destroy native opposition.

Lincoln and Smallpox

President Abraham Lincoln delivered the Gettysburg Address on November 19, 1863. In the days before he gave the famous speech, he reportedly became ill while traveling from Washington, D.C., to Gettysburg, Pennsylvania. Several hours after giving his speech, Lincoln became even sicker. It was a worst-case scenario—the president of the United States had developed smallpox. Luckily, his case was not severe, and he recovered with few noticeable scars. He may have gotten the infection from his son Tad, who also survived the disease. Lincoln may have passed the virus to one of his personal attendants, William H. Johnson, who died from the disease.

Some historians think that Lincoln's doctors may have tried to make his case sound milder than it was so that they would not alarm the American public as the Civil War raged. Others think he may have suffered from *Variola minor*, which is a weaker form of the virus.

A Threat to the Throne

When European royalty was affected by smallpox, the future of entire kingdoms would suddenly be at stake. In 1562, Queen Elizabeth I of England, who was then twenty-nine years old, became ill with smallpox. The Protestant queen was worried that she might die before having a child who could take her place as ruler. If that happened, her Catholic cousin, Mary Queen of Scots, could seize the throne of England and reimpose the Roman faith, which had been rejected by Elizabeth's father, Henry VIII, upon the nation. So for a time, England's political balance of power and religion was threatened by smallpox.

While Queen Elizabeth was sick, her doctors performed red therapy on her. She was wrapped in red clothing and blankets and placed by a raging fire in an attempt to cure the disease. She eventually survived—no thanks to the misguided treatment—but was heavily scarred from the pox. This scarring also resulted in hair loss. For the rest of her life, she wore heavy makeup and wigs to disguise her altered appearance.

Eventually, Queen Elizabeth had her cousin Mary executed. The removal of this rival and threat to her leadership ensured the continuance of her reign and the practice of Protestant religion in England. Elizabeth went on to rule England for forty-five more years. She presided over an incredibly rich period in the nation's history. She fostered a creative and expansive atmosphere that spurred the efforts of literary geniuses, like William Shakespeare and Christopher Marlowe, and explorers such as Sir Walter Raleigh and Sir Francis Drake. The literary, military, and exploratory glories of the Elizabethan Age would establish England's cultural and political dominance over both the Old World and much of the

New World. History would undoubtedly have been different had smallpox killed her when she was only twenty-nine.

Smallpox and the American Revolution

During the 1700s, variolation therapy was common in England. Many American colonists, however, did not embrace the practice as readily as did the British. Laws were sometimes passed in the colonies to prohibit variolation in certain areas. Some people wanted the practice stopped because, even though it helped protect the patient who received the procedure, it could cause the full-blown form of the disease to spread to others. This frightened many people, including the poor, who could not afford the treatment for themselves. As a result of growing public opposition and restrictive anti-variolation laws, fewer colonists had been inoculated against smallpox than had British citizens.

When British soldiers came over to the colonies to quell growing political dissent, they were better protected against smallpox outbreaks than were the colonists. This made it tempting for the British to consider using the disease as a weapon once the Revolutionary War broke out.

George Washington had survived smallpox when he was nineteen years old and had a severely pockmarked face as a result. He originally opposed the idea of variolation for the colonial troops during the American Revolution. He feared it would contribute to a widespread epidemic among the soldiers. However, he eventually heard of the British plot to use smallpox as an early form of germ warfare.

To help prevent this dangerous possibility, General Washington gathered a thousand men who had already suffered and survived the disease. These pockmarked fighters

No. 149. To Col: Christopher Greene. 1. Rhode Island.

Head Quarters Morris Town March 12th 1777.

Sir

You are hereby required immediately to send me an exact return of the state of your Regiment, and to march all the recruits you have, after they get over the small pox, to join the army; leaving a sufficient number of proper Officers to carry on the recruiting Service, who are to follow as fast as they are ready. No pleas, for delay, drawn from the dispersion of the Officers and men, can be admitted. Every command ing officer should know where his inferior officers and these where their recruits are, and should be able to collect them in the most expeditious manner.

You are to remain behind, to complete your Regiment, sending forward your Major, and as circumstances shall permit your Lieutenant Colonel also.

I am Sir. Your most hum.e Serv.t

G Washington.

No. 149. The same to Col: Israel Angell. 2. R. Island

This March 12, 1777, letter from General George Washington to Colonel Christopher Greene seeks information on the health of Greene's troops and an order to send the soldiers under Greene who have recovered from smallpox to join the main army as quickly as possible.

would help level the battlefield between the two armies. They would serve as the forward fighting force that would meet the British head-on and safely absorb any of their attempts to spread deadly contagion. Not long after these developments, George Washington himself became a strong advocate of variolation, and, in 1777, he arranged for all new recruits to undergo it.

Greater Vaccine Safety

Even after Edward Jenner discovered how to use the cowpox virus in an effective smallpox vaccine in 1798, the debate over

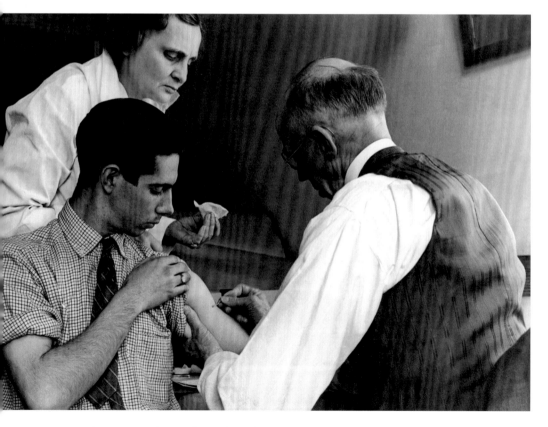

A teenager is vaccinated against smallpox in 1938 by a school doctor. Widespread vaccination was critical in eradicating the disease.

inoculation raged on. Vaccination was widely unregulated. Some methods were not sanitary, or clean. Some people passed the cowpox vaccine from one patient's arm to another, a practice that could spread other infectious agents to patients. As a result, the Vaccination Act was passed in 1898. This act prohibited arm-to-arm transmission for vaccination, which carried a severe risk of transmitting the infectious agent that caused another serious and potentially deadly disease, syphilis.

In 1925, further regulation of vaccines helped make them safer and of higher quality. By the early twentieth century, people understood the importance of vaccination. It did not involve the risks that variolation did, and people recognized that it was a relatively safe and lifesaving procedure. Priests and clergymen spoke out and urged people to have their children vaccinated. Laws were passed to ensure that people received vaccinations in order to keep society safe from this ancient and relentless killer. Eventually, government policies were able to control smallpox, instead of the other way around.

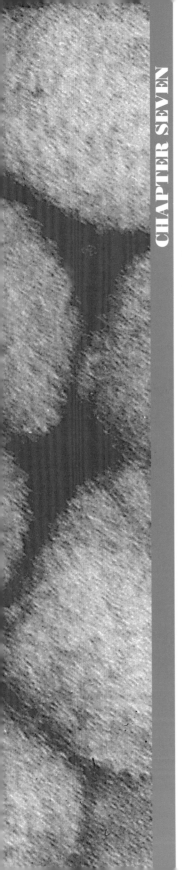

CHAPTER SEVEN

SMALLPOX TODAY

In the war to end smallpox, Edward Jenner's discovery of vaccination was only the first step. Further improvements to Jenner's concepts and techniques would occur in the years following his 1798 discovery. For nearly a century, people risked infections from vaccination needles that were not sterilized, or cleansed of all harmful microorganisms. It was not until the 1890s that sterile, disposable needles were first introduced. This in itself helped save lives and make the smallpox vaccinations more safe and effective.

Louis Pasteur, the now famous chemist and microbiologist, made further breakthroughs in vaccination. He discovered that weakened forms of the actual viruses could be used in vaccines, rather than using preparations from infected animals. So instead of receiving a vaccine containing cowpox, people could instead safely receive a vaccine made of a weakened form of the variola virus that would not cause smallpox.

With modern vaccinations, a person's immune system reacts to the weakened viral or bacterial strain and creates proteins called antibodies. These antibodies recognize and destroy the harmful infectious agent. If the person were to come in contact with a full-strength

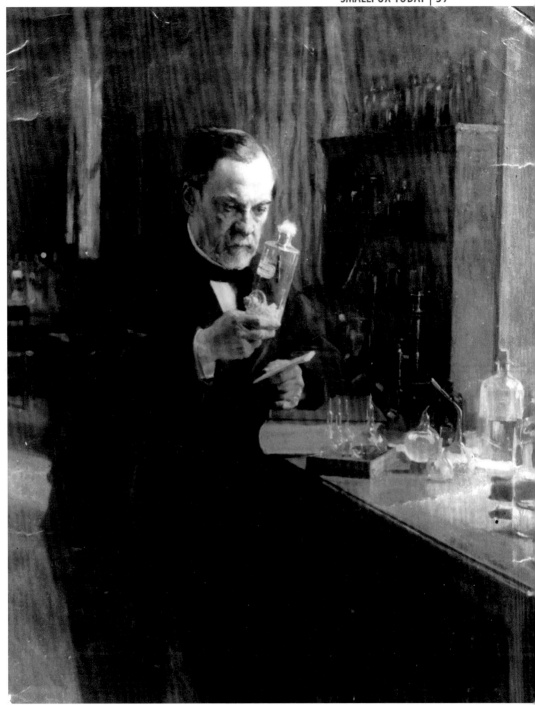

Louis Pasteur played an important role in modernizing vaccines to make them safe and effective.

form of the virus or bacterium, the body would react by relying on a sort of memory of the earlier invasion of the weakened version of the virus and send out the same antibodies used the first time to fight this second invasion. Vaccinations have helped fight against many diseases. Today, bubonic plague, whooping cough, influenza (flu), diphtheria, yellow fever, typhoid, measles, mumps, and hepatitis B are infectious diseases that are now preventable by vaccination.

Today, many people do not even know about smallpox because it has been completely eradicated, or destroyed, as a deadly disease. This remarkable achievement did not happen overnight. Despite vaccination and all we know about how smallpox spreads from person to person, the disease still plagued humankind well into the twentieth century. As recently as the 1930s, fifty thousand Americans a year suffered from smallpox. The last case of the disease in the United States was in Hidalgo, Texas, in 1949.

The World Health Organization Goes to War Against Smallpox

After World War II, the United Nations was formed to help tackle world problems and promote peace, health, and security among all the countries of the world. Within this group, the World Health Organization (WHO) was formed. Its job is to track, monitor, and solve international health issues.

As recently as 1966, an estimated two million people were killed by smallpox worldwide. Cases mainly occurred in African countries south of the Sahara. Many also occurred in Bangladesh, Brazil, India, Indonesia, Nepal, and Pakistan. In many of these parts of the world, vaccines were not easy to get, and many people were not aware of how the disease spread.

WHO resolved to make a final push to eradicate small-pox from the world for good. It would be no easy task, but it was an important effort for the good of all humankind. Even though many people had already been vaccinated and were protected against smallpox, modern travel on airplanes still spread the disease to many places around the world.

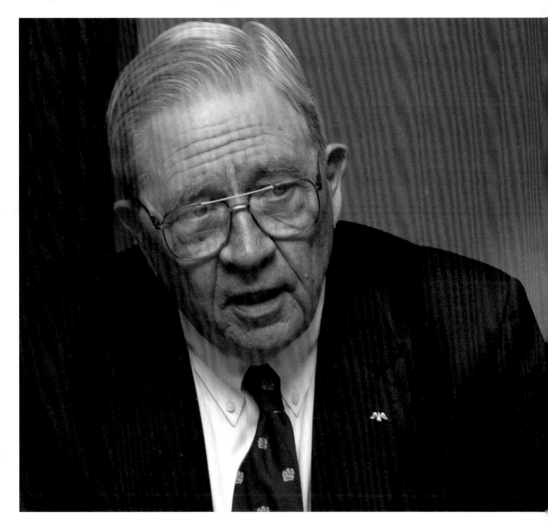

Dr. Donald A. Henderson led the fight to eradicate smallpox worldwide in the 1960s and '70s. Here, he speaks at the University of Arkansas for Medical Sciences on December 11, 2003, about the risk of smallpox being used for the purposes of bioterrorism.

An American doctor, Donald A. Henderson, helped lead WHO's efforts to eliminate smallpox once and for all. Huge vaccination programs in countries that had never had vaccines before were one effort that helped. Another two-step

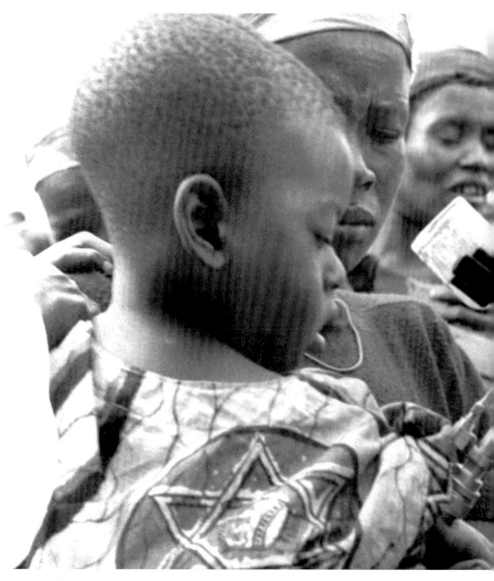

A child in South Cameroon receives a smallpox vaccination as part of a program to eliminate the disease worldwide. The last known case was in 1979.

effort was introduced at the same time. It was called surveillance and containment. In this approach, informational photo pamphlets were passed out around the world so that people from different countries could recognize the symptoms and

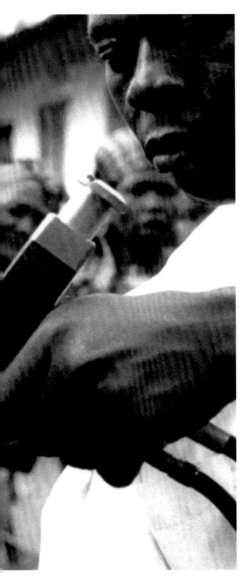

effects of smallpox. Everyone was given the same information and told to alert authorities when these cases were spotted in their region.

As cases were reported, WHO would send fieldworkers to quarantine the affected areas and then vaccinate or revaccinate everyone within a certain radius of the outbreak. This would break the chain of infection and create gaps so that the smallpox virus could not spread to another area. This worldwide effort worked, though very slowly. By 1975, smallpox had disappeared from Asia and South America.

In 1977, a Somalian cook named Ali Maow Maalin was the last known person to have contracted smallpox naturally. He survived the disease. In 1978, one other isolated case of smallpox occurred in a laboratory setting in England, where the variola virus existed only for study by scientists. In this case, an accident in the lab spread the virus to a photographer working in the same building. The woman, Janet Parker, died from smallpox that year. However, the worldwide efforts had succeeded. In 1980, WHO confirmed that the disease had been eradicated and the world was finally free from the scourge of smallpox.

The Future of Smallpox

The United States has been free of smallpox for so long that, since 1972, children no longer receive the vaccination as part of their routine doctor visits. Others who have received vaccinations before this time are no longer immune, however, because the vaccine does not offer lifetime protection.

Has the world seen the last of smallpox? Will this ghastly disease ever plague civilization again? Many officials fear that the disease may again pose a threat if the virus falls into the wrong hands and is used as a biological weapon.

In order to make smallpox vaccines, samples of the virus are needed. Frozen stockpiles of these samples have been stored and safeguarded by the United States in case of an outbreak during which new vaccines would be needed. It is these very stockpiles, however, that could also be used to form the biological weapons that officials fear.

The most troubling evidence of smallpox potentially being used as a biological weapon came in 1998. A man named Ken Alibek told the U.S. government that Russia had

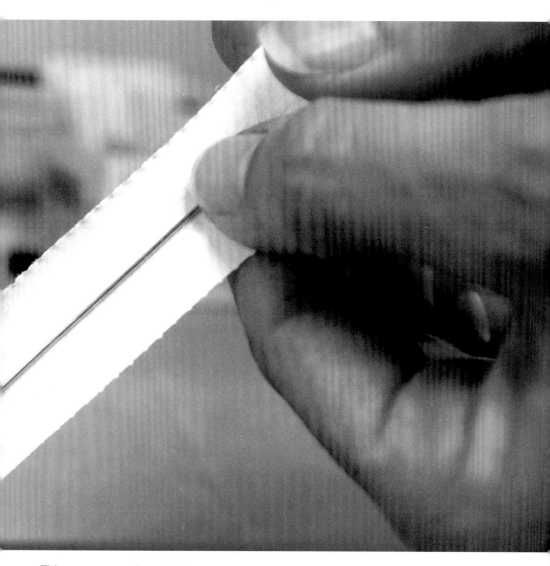

This two-pronged needle is used to give smallpox vaccinations. It was used in a study to test whether existing smallpox vaccines were still effective after being diluted.

made large amounts of smallpox to be used in missiles that could spread the disease around the world. Before immigrating to the United States, Alibek had worked at the Russian company that made these weapons.

As a result of this claim, President Bill Clinton decided to hold onto the U.S. stockpiles of the virus so that they could be used to make future vaccines if necessary. At the time, WHO had been calling for the stockpiles to be destroyed so that they could not cause any further threat to humans. However, the need to hold onto them suddenly became very clear in the wake of Alibek's disclosure.

As of 2001, the United States had enough smallpox vaccine to immunize between six and fifteen million people. After the terrorist attacks of September 11, 2001, President George W. Bush planned to produce enough smallpox vaccine to immunize the entire country. Since that time, researchers discovered that existing vaccines would be just as effective if they are diluted, or made less concentrated. That would help labs quickly create five times as many vaccines from the already existing stockpiles. Currently, the United States has enough smallpox vaccines to protect everyone in the United States. Both the Department of Defense, as well as the Centers for Disease Control and Prevention (CDC), have produced smallpox vaccine stockpiles in case they are needed in the future.

By March 2007, about 1.2 million military personnel and health care workers had already received smallpox vaccinations. If a future outbreak were to occur, these people would need to be protected first in order to respond to a smallpox national security and health care emergency. It would also free up the remaining vaccination stockpile for the rest of the population.

The Death of a Killer?

If there is one person responsible for keeping the world free of smallpox, it's Edward Jenner. His discovery of vaccination helped protect the world against the most deadly killer civilization has ever known. Any future threat of smallpox can likely be halted by vaccination as well.

Billions of people have died from smallpox. It is terrifying to think that this dreaded disease may purposefully be inflicted on the world through the murderous cruelty of others. But we can also look on the bright side. Unlike the billions of people who died of the disease in the past, we have modern medicine on our side. We are fortunate to live in a time when we already have a cure for the future smallpox threats that we might face. We have seen the successful eradication of a disease that has attacked and disrupted civilization for thousands of years. Optimistically, smallpox will never again return to wreak havoc on our families, our communities, our governments and nations, and our very lives. We can only hope that smallpox has been banished from our world forever.

TEN GREAT QUESTIONS to ask a DOCTOR

1 Has smallpox disappeared entirely worldwide?

2 Am I likely to be exposed to the variola virus where I live?

3 Can I be infected with the variola virus just by brushing against someone who is infected or touching a doorknob he or she has touched?

4 If I have been exposed to the variola virus, is there any use in receiving a vaccination soon after exposure?

5 When do you know that a person infected with the variola virus is no longer contagious?

6 At what age should someone receive the smallpox vaccination?

7 Does the vaccine provide lifelong protection, or are booster shots necessary after being inoculated against smallpox?

8 How secure from theft are laboratory samples of the variola virus?

9 If there were an outbreak of smallpox, is there enough vaccine stockpiled to protect everyone in the country?

10 What is the modern mortality rate for those infected with the variola virus?

GLOSSARY

contagious Easily spread from person to person.

diluted Made weaker or thinner by adding water or another liquid.

endemic Describing something that is commonly found among a population or geographic area.

epidemic A new outbreak (i.e., beyond normal levels) of a disease that affects a population.

eradicate To completely destroy or put an end to something.

immune system The body's defenses that recognize and fight agents of infectious disease.

immunity The ability of an organism to resist, protect against, and/or fight infection.

immunology The study of the cells and responses of the immune system.

infectious Likely to be transmitted from person to person; contagious.

inoculation The introduction of an infectious agent into the body for the purpose of generating immunity.

mutation A change in the genetic information of an organism or infectious agent.

outbreak The sudden or violent start of something.

stockpile A large collection of goods or materials that may be used in case of emergency or time of shortage.

pandemic An outbreak that is widespread around a geographic region or around the world.

pockmark A permanent scar on the skin following infection by smallpox or other pox diseases.

pustule A pus-filled, pimplelike blister.

quarantine The period of time when a contagious person is placed in isolation during a disease outbreak.

sterilized Cleaned completely, so there is no contamination with infectious agents.

vaccination The practice of giving a foreign substance, such as a weakened form of a virus, to someone to generate immunity to an infectious agent.

variolation The practice of giving someone a weaker form of the smallpox virus in order to prevent infection with the variola virus and development of smallpox.

virus A microscopic infectious agent that uses other living cells to replicate; many viruses cause disease.

FOR MORE INFORMATION

American Council on Science and Health
1995 Broadway, Second Floor
New York, NY 10023-5860
(212) 362-7044
Web site: http://www.acsh.org
The American Council on Science and Health is a
group of consumer education advocates that
includes doctors, scientists, and policy makers.

American Public Health Association
800 I Street NW
Washington, DC 20001
(202) 777-2742
Web site: http://www.apha.org
The American Public Health Association is an
organization of health professionals dedicated to
improving public health.

Centers for Disease Control and Prevention
1600 Clifton Road
Atlanta, GA 30333
(800) 232-4636
Web site: http://www.cdc.gov
The Centers for Disease Control and Prevention is
an organization that provides the public with
reliable information about disease and health-
related topics.

Health Canada
A.L. 0904A
Ottawa, ON K1A 0K9
Canada

(613) 957-2991
Web site: http://www.hc-sc.gc.ca
Health Canada is a government department that helps
    Canadians maintain and improve their health.

Public Health Agency of Canada
1015 Arlington Street
Winnipeg, MB R3E3R2
Canada
(204) 789-2000
Web site: http://www.phac-aspc.gc.ca
The Public Health Agency of Canada is a government orga-
    nization that promotes health and helps people to prevent
    and control diseases, injuries, and infections.

World Health Organization
Avenue Appia 20
1211 Geneva 27
Switzerland
Phone: + 41 22 791 21 11
Web site: http://www.who.int/en
The World Health Organization is part of the United Nations.
    It provides health leadership for the world and monitors
    health trends worldwide.

Web Sites

Due to the changing nature of Internet links, Rosen
Publishing has developed an online list of Web sites related
to the subject of this book. This site is updated regularly.
Please use this link to access this list:

http://www.rosenlinks.com/epi/smal

FOR FURTHER READING

Arnold, Nick. *Deadly Diseases and Microscopic Monsters*. New York, NY: Scholastic, 2009.

Ballard, Edward. *On Vaccinations*. Charleston, SC: BiblioBazaar, 2008.

Brownlee, Christen. *Cute, Furry, and Deadly: Diseases You Can Catch from Your Pet*. New York, NY: Children's Press, 2007.

Dendy, Leslie, and Mel Boring. *Guinea Pig Scientists: Bold Self-Experimenters in Science and Medicine*. New York, NY: Henry Holt and Co., 2005.

Emmeluth, Donald. *Plague* (Deadly Diseases and Epidemics). New York, NY: Chelsea House Publications, 2005.

Farrell, Jeanette. *Invisible Enemies: Stories of Infectious Disease*. New York, NY: FSG, 2005.

Finer, Kim. *Smallpox* (Deadly Diseases and Epidemics). New York, NY: Facts on File, 2004.

Friedlander, Mark P., Jr. *Outbreak: Disease Detectives at Work*. Minneapolis, MN: Twenty-First Century Books, 2009.

Glynn, Ian, and Jenifer Glynn. *The Life and Death of Smallpox*. New York, NY: Cambridge University Press, 2004.

Henderson, D. A. *Smallpox: The Death of a Disease: The Inside Story of Eradicating a Worldwide Killer*. Amherst, NY: Prometheus Books, 2009.

Jenner, Edward. *On Vaccination Against Smallpox*. Gloucester, England: Dodo Press, 2009.

Kajelle, Marylou Morano. *Louis Pasteur: Fighter Against Infectious Disease*. New York, NY: Mitchell Lane Publishers, 2005.

Mara, Will. *Smallpox* (Outbreak). New York, NY: Children's Press, 2007.

Ollhoff, Jim. *Smallpox* (A History of Germs). Edina, MN: ABDO Publishing Company, 2009.

Rodriquez, Ana Maria. *Edward Jenner: Conqueror of Smallpox*. Berkeley Heights, NJ: Enslow Publishers, 2006.

Saffer, Barbara. *Smallpox* (Diseases and Disorders). Chicago, IL: Lucent Books, 2003.

True Peters, Stephanie. *Smallpox in the New World* (Epidemic!). Tarrytown, NY: Marshall Cavendish Children's Books, 2004.

Walker, Richard. *Epidemics and Plagues*. Boston, MA: Kingfisher, 2007.

BIBLIOGRAPHY

Broad, William J. "Smallpox: The Once and Future Scourge?" June 15, 1999. Retrieved June 28, 2009 (http://www.nytimes.com/1999/06/15/science/smallpox-the-once-and-future-scourge.html).

Bryner, Jeanna. "Did Abe Lincoln Have Smallpox?" MSNBC.com, May 17, 2007. Retrieved June 2009 (http://www.msnbc.msn.com/id/18727435).

Diamond, Jared. *Guns, Germs, and Steel: The Fates of Human Societies*. New York, NY: W. W. Norton & Company, 2005.

Dunlap, David W. "Smallpox Hospital on Roosevelt Island Crumbles." *New York Times*, January 4, 2008. Retrieved July 18, 2009 (http://cityroom.blogs.nytimes.com/2008/01/04/smallpox-hospital-on-roosevelt-island-crumbles).

Fenn, Elizabeth A. *Pox Americana: The Great Smallpox Epidemic of 1775–82*. New York, NY: Hill and Wang, 2001.

Fenner, Frank, et al. *Smallpox and Its Eradication*. Geneva, Switzerland: World Health Organization, 1988.

Glynn, Ian, and Jenifer Glynn. *The Life and Death of Smallpox*. New York, NY: Cambridge University Press, 2004.

History Channel. *History's Mysteries: Smallpox* (DVD). New York, NY: A&E Television Network, 2002.

Hopkins, Donald R. *The Greatest Killer: Smallpox in History*. Chicago, IL: University of Chicago Press, 2002.

Koplow, David. *Smallpox: The Fight to Eradicate a Global Scourge*. Berkeley, CA: University of California Press, 2003.

Mann, Charles C. *1491: New Revelations of the Americas Before Columbus*. New York, NY: Vintage Books, 2006.

Marrin, Albert. *Dr. Jenner and the Speckled Monster*. New York, NY: Dutton Children's Books, 2002.

Oldstone, Michael B. *Viruses, Plagues, and History*. New York, NY: Oxford University Press, 1998.

Ridgway, Tom. *Smallpox* (Epidemics: Deadly Diseases Through History). New York, NY: Rosen Publishing Group, 2001.

Tandon, Henry. *"Smallpox Hospital."* Roosevelt Island Historical Society, 2000. Retrieved July 18, 2009 (http://www.correctionhistory.org/rooseveltisland/html/rooseveltislandtour_smallpox.html).

Ward, Geoffrey C. *The West: An Illustrated History*. Boston, MA: Little, Brown and Company, 1996.

INDEX

About the Author

Adam Furgang has written several books for Rosen Publishing on topics such as the environment and technology. He is a writer and artist who has always had a lifelong interest and appreciation for all things scientific.

Photo Credits

Front cover (left), back cover (right) © www.istockphoto.com/adisa; front cover (right), back cover (left), pp. 6, 12, 14, 24, 33, 41, 49, 58, 62–63, 69, 71, 73, 75, 77 CDC; pp. 4–5 Getty Images; p. 7 Murphy/Whitfield/Centers for Disease Control and Prevention/Photo Researchers, Inc.; pp. 8–9 James Gathany/CDC; p. 16 Courtesy of WHO; p. 18 © Jack Novak/SuperStock; pp. 20–21 © North Wind Picture Archives/Alamy; p. 25 Edward Gooch/ Hulton Archive/Getty Images; pp. 29, 59 Hulton Archive/Getty Images; pp. 30, 38–39, 45 Courtesy of the National Library of Medicine; p. 31 SSPL/Getty Images; pp. 34–35 © The Print Collector/Alamy; pp. 36 Library of Congress Prints and Photographs Division; pp. 42–43 Musee des Beaux-Arts, Lyon, France/The Bridgeman Art Library/Getty Images; pp. 46–47 The New York Public Library/Art Resource, NY (detail of an original stereoscopic view); p. 50 Bibliotheque de L'Arsenal, Paris, France/ The Bridgeman Art Library/Getty Images; p. 51 Library of Congress Rare Book and Special Collections Division; p. 55 Library of Congress Manuscript Division; p. 56 FPG/Hulton Archive/Getty Images; p. 61 © AP Images; pp. 64–65 Justin Sullivan/Getty Images.

Designer: Sam Zavieh; Photo Researcher: Cindy Reiman